Everyday Mindfulness:

10 Quick Practices to Reduce Stress & Find Peace

Contents

Chapter 1: Introduction to Mindfulness

What is Mindfulness?

Mindfulness is one of those words that seems to be everywhere these days, but what does it actually mean? Simply put, mindfulness is the practice of bringing your full attention to the present moment, without judgment. Imagine it as a mental "pause button," a way to set down the endless to-do lists, worries, and distractions—if only for a moment. When we're mindful, we're fully here, noticing what's happening around us and within us. We're not caught up in the past or rushing into the future.

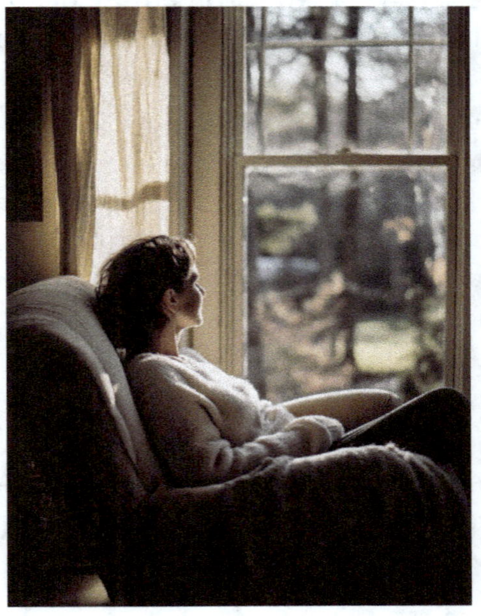

Think of mindfulness as a chance to reconnect with yourself in a world that often feels chaotic and overwhelming. It's a moment to breathe, to check in, and to refresh. And the best part? You don't need any special skills or hours of free time to practice it. Mindfulness is accessible to everyone, and with some simple tools, you can start experiencing its benefits right away.

Why Start Now?

So, why even bother with mindfulness? The truth is, many of us are looking for ways to manage stress, stay focused, and feel a little more balanced. Mindfulness has been shown to help with all of this. Science backs it up — mindfulness can lower stress, improve focus, and even boost our mental health. But beyond the science, there's something deeply fulfilling about just being fully present, even if only for a few minutes each day.

If you're like most people, you might often feel overwhelmed or on autopilot. Maybe you're rushing from one thing to the next, or maybe you're distracted by a hundred different thoughts. Mindfulness offers an antidote to this busy way of living. It gives us permission to slow down and find peace in the here and now, without feeling pressured to "do" anything.

And here's some good news: you don't need to commit hours to mindfulness to feel a difference. Small, consistent steps — like the ones we'll explore in this book — can add up to a big impact over time.

Mindfulness Myths (and Real Truths)

If you're new to mindfulness, you might have heard a few things that sound intimidating. Let's bust a few common myths and replace them with some truths:

- **Myth #1**: Mindfulness means "emptying" your mind.
  Truth: Mindfulness isn't about clearing your mind or having zero thoughts (thank goodness!). It's more about noticing your thoughts and letting them be there without getting swept away.
- **Myth #2**: You need a quiet, peaceful space to practice.
  Truth: While a calm environment can help, mindfulness can be practiced anywhere—at your desk, on the bus, or even in the middle of a busy day. All you need is a few moments of focus.

- **Myth #3**: Mindfulness takes hours of practice.
  Truth: A few minutes can make a difference. You don't have to dedicate large chunks of time to see results. Mindfulness is about quality, not quantity.

By clearing up these myths, we hope you feel encouraged to start. Mindfulness is a skill that anyone can learn and use, no matter how busy life gets.

The Science Behind Mindfulness

(Without the Jargon)

Here's the quick version: mindfulness actually changes the brain in ways that help us feel calmer and more in control. When we practice mindfulness, we're engaging parts of the brain that help us manage emotions, while reducing activity in areas associated with stress. For example, mindfulness has been shown to lower blood pressure and reduce levels of the stress hormone cortisol.

If you're someone who likes knowing the "why" behind things, you can rest assured that mindfulness is backed by solid research. But for now, all you really need to know is that this simple practice works — and it can help you feel more balanced and grounded in your daily life.

Mini-Reflection: Take a moment to ask yourself, "How often do I feel like I'm just going through the motions?" Imagine if you could feel more present, more connected, and even a little bit more at peace — even for just a few moments a day. This is what mindfulness can offer.

The Beginner's Mindset

As you dive into mindfulness, one of the most helpful things you can bring is a beginner's mindset. What does that mean? A beginner's mindset is about approaching each practice with curiosity, letting go of any expectations or pressure to get it "right." There's no perfect way to be mindful, and everyone's experience is a bit different.

Starting out, you might feel awkward or even a little silly, and that's perfectly okay! Remember, mindfulness is a journey, not a destination. Give yourself permission to learn and explore, just as you would with any new skill. And if things feel messy or challenging at times, that's all part of the process.

First Simple Exercise: Breathing in Awareness

Let's get started with a small taste of mindfulness. This exercise is simple but powerful, and you can come back to it whenever you need a moment of calm.

1. **Find a comfortable seat**. Sit in a way that feels easy, whether on a chair, the floor, or wherever you are.
2. **Close your eyes if you feel comfortable**. This isn't necessary, but it can help you focus.
3. **Take a deep breath in**. Notice how the air feels as it enters your nose and fills your lungs. Then let it out slowly.
4. **Repeat for a few breaths**. As you breathe in, say silently to yourself, "Breathing in." As you breathe out, think, "Breathing out."
5. **Check in with yourself**. After a few breaths, pause and notice: Do you feel any different? Is there a sense of calm, or maybe a bit of tension? Either way is fine; the goal is simply to notice.

This exercise might only take a minute, but it's a small step toward cultivating mindfulness. Try it whenever you need a quick mental reset—on a busy day, before a big meeting, or even while waiting in line.

What You'll Gain from This Book

If this quick practice felt helpful, you're on the right path. In the next chapters, we'll explore more ways to bring mindfulness into everyday moments—whether you're at home, at work, or on the go. The exercises will be short, practical, and designed to fit into even the busiest of days.

Remember, mindfulness is a tool that you can carry with you wherever you go. Each chapter will add a new layer to this tool, helping you build a sense of calm and focus in your daily life.

Let's get started!

Chapter 2: Setting Up for Success

Creating Space for Mindfulness

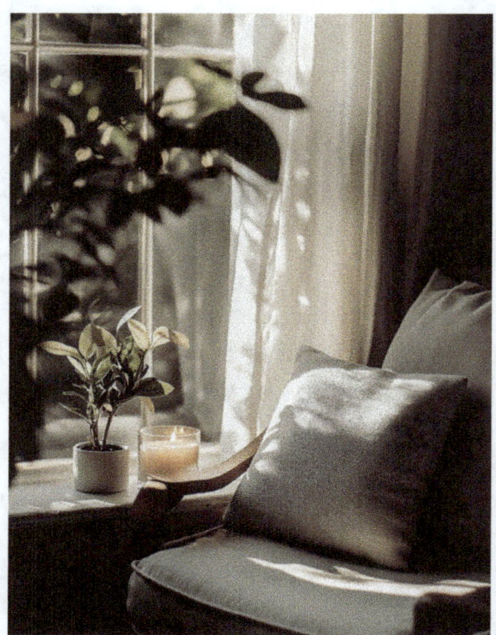

Starting any new practice can feel a bit overwhelming, especially when life is already busy. The good news is that mindfulness doesn't require big changes to your routine or a special setup. In fact, one of the best things about mindfulness is that you can practice it anytime, anywhere. But to make it feel like a lasting habit, creating a small space and time for mindfulness can make all the difference.

Physical Space: Make It Yours

Designate a spot in your home where you feel comfortable practicing mindfulness, even if it's just a small corner. This could be a cosy chair, a favourite nook by a window, or even a spot on the floor with a pillow. Try to make it inviting, perhaps with a candle, a small plant, or anything that brings you a sense of calm.

Having this space, however small, signals to your mind, "This is my time to slow down." And remember, while a designated space can be helpful, it's absolutely not essential. Mindfulness can happen wherever you are.

Mental Space: Finding Focus Amidst Chaos

Creating space mentally can be the real challenge, especially when your mind is full of thoughts. Don't worry about trying to "clear your mind" (that's actually impossible!). Instead, aim to set aside a few minutes where you can bring your focus inward, even if distractions are present.

Here's a helpful approach: take a few seconds before you start each practice to mentally acknowledge any worries or to-dos. Tell yourself, "For the next few minutes, I'm putting everything else on hold. It will still be there afterward." This small mental shift can help you settle into mindfulness more easily.

Mindfulness Goals: Start Small and Stay Realistic

When we start something new, it's easy to set big, ambitious goals. But with mindfulness, sometimes less is more. Rather than aiming for perfection, try setting a few small, achievable goals. For example, you might start by committing to just five minutes of mindfulness a day, or practicing a simple breathing exercise each morning before your day gets busy.

A Few Goal Ideas:

- **Daily Practice**: Aim for a few minutes of mindfulness each day. Even a short session can make a difference.

- **Being Present in Daily Tasks**: Choose one daily activity, like brushing your teeth or washing dishes, and practice being fully present for it.
- **Checking In Weekly**: Once a week, reflect on your mindfulness journey. Ask yourself, "How did it feel to practice mindfulness this week? What did I notice?"

Keeping goals small and approachable makes it easier to build mindfulness into your life without it feeling like a chore. The more realistic and specific your goals, the more likely they'll become habits.

Getting Comfortable with the Process

One thing that can help beginners is to let go of expectations. Starting a mindfulness practice is a bit like learning to play an instrument. You wouldn't expect yourself to be a pro musician after one lesson, right? The same goes for mindfulness. There might be days when it feels easy and days when it feels like nothing's working—and that's okay.

Patience and Self-Compassion

Give yourself permission to feel however you feel. Some days you might feel more focused, and other days you might find it hard to sit still. Mindfulness is about observing what's happening in the moment, without adding judgment. So if you feel restless, just notice it and let it be. Practicing self-compassion (or kindness toward yourself) can make a huge difference in how you experience mindfulness.

A Simple Mindfulness Routine to Start

To get the most out of this book, let's create a simple starting routine. This will help you ease into the practice without feeling overwhelmed. Here's a routine you can try each day, for as little or as much time as you have.

The Daily Mindful Minute:

1. **Settle In**: Find your designated spot, or simply sit wherever you are.
2. **Take a Deep Breath**: Breathe in deeply through your nose, and slowly release it through your mouth.
3. **Focus on Your Breath**: For the next minute, focus on each breath you take. Notice the feeling of the air entering and leaving your body. If your mind wanders, gently bring it back to your breath.
4. **Wrap Up with Gratitude**: After your minute is up, think of one thing you're grateful for in that moment. It could be anything, big or small. This small act of gratitude can be a powerful way to end your practice.

This one-minute practice is a wonderful way to begin. The simplicity of focusing on your breath for just a minute can help set the tone for your day or provide a calming reset whenever you need it.

Building a Sustainable Mindfulness Practice

Once you've established a daily minute of mindfulness, you may want to expand your practice. But remember, mindfulness is all about what works for you. If you find that one minute is enough, that's perfectly fine. You don't need to feel pressured to increase your practice if it's not something you feel ready for.

Finding Balance

Balance is key. Rather than seeing mindfulness as something extra on your to-do list, try to view it as a moment for yourself. Think of it as your chance to check in, recharge, and take a break from everything else.

You might decide to gradually add more time as you feel comfortable, but there's no rush. The goal is to make mindfulness feel like a natural part of your life, not another obligation.

Remember: There's No "Right" Way

As you set up your mindfulness practice, it's helpful to remember that there's no "perfect" way to do this. Mindfulness isn't about getting it "right" — it's about exploring and experiencing each moment as it comes.

If your mind wanders a lot, that's normal. If you get frustrated, that's also normal. Let yourself approach mindfulness with a sense of curiosity. You're not trying to achieve a specific outcome. Instead, you're giving yourself the space to be exactly as you are.

Ending the Chapter with Encouragement

Starting a mindfulness journey is an amazing act of self-care. You're giving yourself a gift: a chance to find calm, clarity, and balance in a busy world. As you continue through this book, keep this sense of curiosity and kindness with you.

Remember, mindfulness isn't a destination; it's a way of being. And each small step you take—whether it's a one-minute breathing exercise or simply noticing the world around you—brings you closer to the peace and presence you're looking for.

Let's keep going.

Chapter 3: The Power of the Breath

Breathing Basics: Why Breath Matters

Our breath is something we often take for granted. It's always there, quietly working in the background. But did you know that our breath is one of the most powerful tools we have for calming the mind and body? When we breathe mindfully, we can change our stress levels, our focus, and even our mood within just a few moments.

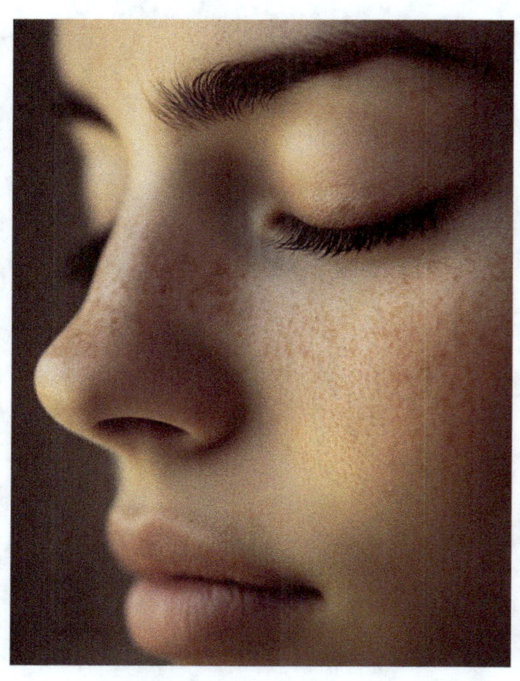

Breathing is something we can control, and it's available to us wherever we are. When we intentionally focus on our breath, it helps us anchor into the present moment. This is why mindfulness often starts with breathing—it's the simplest way to bring our attention to *right here, right now*. The more we connect with our breath, the more we can find a sense of calm and clarity in our daily lives.

In this chapter, we'll explore a few basic breathing techniques that you can use anytime you need a mental reset, feel overwhelmed, or just want a moment to connect with yourself.

Easy Breathing Techniques for Everyday Moments

Here are a few simple breathing exercises you can try. Each one is designed to be quick, effective, and accessible for beginners. Try them out and see which ones work best for you.

1. Deep Belly Breathing

This exercise helps calm your nervous system and reduce stress.

1. **Sit or lie down comfortably**: Place one hand on your belly and one on your chest.
2. **Inhale deeply through your nose**: As you breathe in, try to send the air down to your belly, so the hand on your belly rises more than the one on your chest.
3. **Exhale slowly through your mouth**: Gently push all the air out, noticing your belly fall.
4. **Repeat for a few breaths**: Focus on the rise and fall of your belly, letting each breath be slow and deep.

This type of deep breathing can be a great way to ground yourself in moments of stress or anxiety. When you focus on filling your belly with each breath, it signals your body to relax and slows down your heart rate.

2. Counting Breath

If your mind is racing, this exercise can help you focus.

1. **Start with a deep inhale**: Breathe in through your nose for a slow count of 4.
2. **Hold for a count of 4**: Pause your breath at the top.
3. **Exhale for a count of 4**: Breathe out fully, slowly, to a count of 4.

4. **Repeat**: You can increase or decrease the count to find a
    rhythm that feels comfortable.

This exercise is sometimes called "box breathing" because of the
four-part structure. It's especially helpful if you feel scattered or
need to bring your mind into focus quickly.

3. Three-Part Breath (Complete Breath)

This exercise teaches you to fully expand your lungs, making
each breath feel refreshing.

1. **Inhale deeply through your nose**: As you breathe in, fill the
    lower part of your lungs (your belly), then the middle (your
    ribcage), and finally the upper part (your chest).
2. **Exhale slowly**: Reverse the process, letting the air out from
    your chest, then your ribcage, and finally your belly.
3. **Repeat for a few breaths**: Feel the breath move smoothly
    through each "part" of your lungs.

The Three-Part Breath is a great way to bring a sense of fullness
and flow to your breathing. It can be particularly relaxing when
you feel tightness in your chest or upper body.

4. The Sighing Breath

This exercise is perfect for releasing tension or frustration.

1. Inhale deeply through your nose: Breathe in fully.
2. **Exhale through your mouth with a sigh**: Let out a soft,
    audible sigh as you release your breath.
3. **Repeat**: Try this for a few breaths, noticing how each sigh
    releases tension.

The sighing breath is a simple yet effective way to let go of
stress, especially if you're feeling a buildup of emotions. It's a
gentle reminder to release what's weighing on you, even if just
for a moment.

Real-Life Applications: When to Use These Techniques

Now that you have a few breathing exercises to try, let's talk about when you can use them. Remember, these are meant to be easy tools that fit into your day, whether you're at home, work, or out and about. Here are some everyday scenarios where mindful breathing can be especially helpful:

- **Before a Big Meeting or Event**: Taking a few deep belly breaths or doing a quick counting breath can help you centre yourself, releasing nervous energy and boosting focus.
- **During a Stressful Moment**: If you're in the middle of a hectic day or dealing with something stressful, try the sighing breath to release tension.
- **At the End of the Day**: Use the three-part breath as a way to unwind. As you let each breath move through your body, you're giving yourself permission to relax.
- **Whenever You Need a Reset**: These breathing exercises are here for you anytime you feel the need to pause, slow down, or connect with yourself.

Building the Habit of Breath Awareness

Breath awareness doesn't have to be something you only do during a formal practice. In fact, the more you bring it into daily life, the more natural it becomes. Here are a few tips for building a habit of mindful breathing:

1. **Set Reminders**: Use small reminders throughout the day—a Post-it on your desk, a notification on your phone, or pairing it with an existing routine like brushing your teeth or drinking water.
2. **Check in with Your Breath**: Whenever you remember, pause and notice your breath. Is it shallow? Deep? Fast or slow? This simple check-in can help you reset.

3. **Be Kind to Yourself**: If you forget to breathe mindfully, don't
    worry! Just bring your attention back to it whenever you can.

Breath Awareness as a Lifelong Tool

Mindful breathing isn't just a practice—it's a tool you can rely
on throughout your life. With time, these exercises become
something you can turn to naturally, like a familiar friend,
whenever you need support.

Remember, there's no "perfect" way to breathe mindfully. Some
days you may feel deeply connected to your breath, and other
days it may feel harder to focus. That's okay! The goal is simply
to notice, be present, and allow each breath to bring you back to
this moment.

Chapter Reflection: Connecting with Your Breath

As you finish this chapter, take a moment to reflect on what you
experienced with these exercises. How did it feel to focus on
your breath? Did any of the techniques feel particularly helpful
or soothing?

If you'd like, write down a few thoughts about your experience
with mindful breathing. This can help you remember which
exercises resonate most and give you something to look back on
as you continue your journey.

Chapter 4: Cultivating Present-Moment Awareness

What it Means to Be Present

"Being present" is one of those phrases we hear a lot, but what

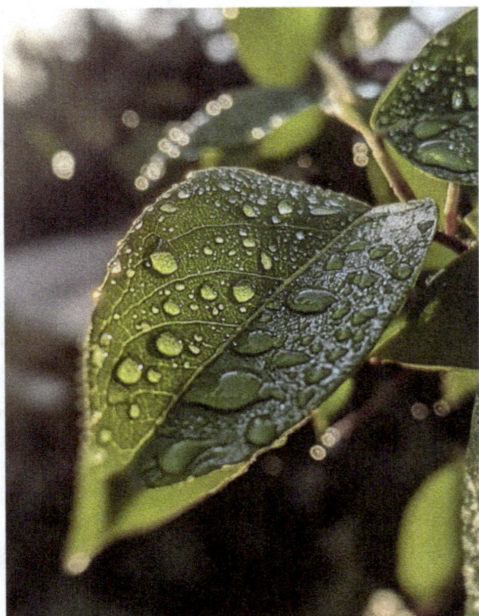

does it actually mean? At its core, being present is simply the act of fully experiencing each moment as it comes. It means noticing what's happening around you and within you, without getting caught up in worries about the past or future.

Think of how many times a day you're physically in one place but your mind is somewhere else—replaying a conversation, worrying about tomorrow, or checking off your mental to-do list. It's easy to get swept away in thoughts, but when we bring our attention to the present, we're choosing to step out of that mental rush and engage more deeply with life.

Mindfulness is all about cultivating this kind of presence. By learning to bring our attention back to the here and now, we can experience life more fully, even in the simplest moments. In this chapter, we'll explore a few easy ways to practice present-moment awareness and make it a natural part of your day.

Mindful Observation Exercises

Below are a few exercises to help you start building present-moment awareness. These practices are short, practical, and designed to fit into daily life. Try them out and see which ones resonate with you.

1. The Five Senses Check-In

This exercise uses your five senses to ground you in the present moment. It's simple, quick, and effective for when you need a mindful pause.

1. **Pause and take a deep breath**: Allow yourself to settle for a moment.
2. **Notice five things you can see**: Look around and take in your surroundings. Notice colours, shapes, and details.
3. **Notice four things you can touch**: Feel the texture of your clothing, the surface you're sitting on, or an object nearby.
4. **Notice three things you can hear**: Listen for sounds you might not usually notice—birds outside, a ticking clock, or even silence.
5. **Notice two things you can smell**: Take a moment to notice any scents around you, like the smell of coffee or fresh air.
6. **Notice one thing you can taste**: If you have a drink or food nearby, take a small sip or bite and really savour it.

This quick check-in is an easy way to bring yourself back to the present, using your senses to reconnect with the world around you.

2. Mindful Walking

Walking is something we do all the time, often without thinking. Mindful walking helps us turn this routine action into a moment of calm and focus.

1. **Start by walking slowly**: If possible, walk somewhere quiet, like a park or hallway. Focus on each step.
2. **Notice the feeling in your feet**: Pay attention to how each foot feels as it lifts, moves forward, and touches the ground.
3. **Observe your breath**: Breathe naturally and notice how your breath aligns with your steps.
4. **Engage your senses**: Take in your surroundings as you walk. Notice colours, sounds, or the feeling of air on your skin.

Mindful walking can be a calming way to reset, especially if you're feeling tense or have been sitting for a while. Even a short, mindful walk can bring a sense of clarity and calm to your day.

3. The One-Minute Pause

This exercise is great for those moments when you feel overwhelmed or need a mental break. It's a simple way to check in with yourself and find balance.

1. **Pause for one minute**: Wherever you are, stop and take a deep breath.
2. **Notice your body**: Take a few seconds to scan your body. Are there any areas of tension? Notice how your body feels in this moment.
3. **Observe your surroundings**: Look around and notice one or two things you hadn't noticed before.
4. **Take one more deep breath**: End with a deep breath and continue with your day.

The One-Minute Pause is like pressing a "reset" button. It reminds you to take a moment for yourself and return to your day with fresh energy.

Building the Habit of Awareness

As you try these exercises, remember that present-moment awareness is something you can practice anywhere. It's about paying attention to what's happening around you without needing anything to change.

Tips for Practicing Awareness Daily:

1. **Pair Awareness with Daily Routines**: Try choosing a few moments throughout your day to practice awareness. For example, when brushing your teeth, try focusing entirely on the sensations involved—the feel of the brush, the taste of the toothpaste, and the sound of the water.
2. **Set Reminders**: Use gentle reminders throughout your day, like a phone notification or a small note on your desk, to pause and come back to the present.
3. **Accept Distractions**: It's natural for your mind to wander, especially at first. When it does, just gently guide your focus back to the present moment without frustration. Over time, this will become easier.

The Benefits of Present-Moment Awareness

You might be wondering, "Why is it so important to stay present?" When we're truly present, we often feel more at ease, more aware, and more connected. Research has shown that present-moment awareness can reduce stress, increase happiness, and improve overall well-being.

When you're fully engaged with what's happening right now, you're not stuck in past regrets or future worries. You're just here, experiencing life as it unfolds. This presence is where mindfulness shines—it's not about escaping reality but about connecting more deeply with it.

Everyday Presence: Building Awareness into Daily Life

Present-moment awareness doesn't require special skills or extra time. Here are a few ways to bring more presence into your day-to-day routine:

- **When Eating**: Take a moment to appreciate the colours, textures, and flavours of your food. Eating mindfully can enhance enjoyment and help you feel more connected to the experience.
- **When Listening to Others**: Practice listening mindfully by focusing on what the person is saying without planning your response. This can help you feel more connected to others and improve relationships.
- **When Using Technology**: Try putting away your phone or turning off screens for a few moments each day. This small act can create more space for awareness and help reduce mental clutter.

Practicing Awareness in Challenging Moments

Present-moment awareness can be particularly helpful during stressful times. When you're feeling overwhelmed or frustrated, try grounding yourself with one of the exercises from earlier in the chapter. Whether it's taking a one-minute pause or a mindful walk, these small practices remind you that you have control over where your attention goes.

If you can stay present even during challenging moments, you'll likely feel more equipped to handle stress and find balance. It's not about ignoring difficulties but about choosing to face them with a calm, grounded mind.

Chapter Reflection: Living in the Now

As you wrap up this chapter, take a moment to think on how it felt to practice present-moment awareness. Did you notice anything new or surprising about your surroundings? Were there moments when you felt more connected or calm?

Jot down a few thoughts on your experience. Building present-moment awareness is like planting seeds — they grow with time and gentle attention. The more you practice, the easier it becomes to be fully present and embrace life as it unfolds.

Chapter 5: Mindfulness at Home and Work

Why Mindfulness Matters in Everyday Routines

Life doesn't pause when we're at home or work—if anything, it often feels busier. But the great thing about mindfulness is that it can fit into these everyday spaces, helping us find small moments of calm and clarity no matter where we are. Whether you're washing dishes, responding to emails, or in the middle of a big meeting, bringing mindfulness into your daily routines can make everything feel a little more manageable and meaningful.

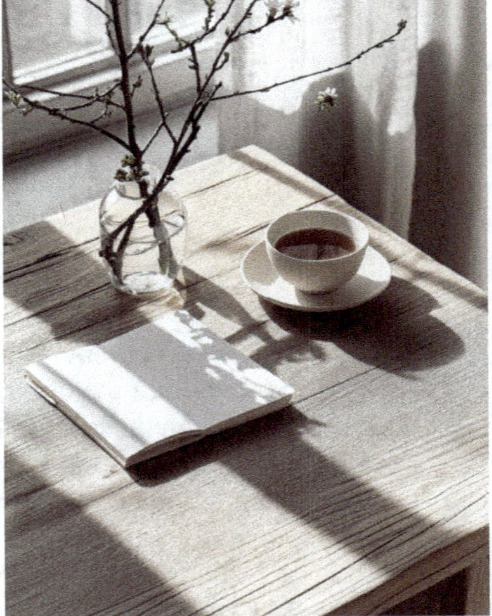

In this chapter, we'll look at simple ways to practice mindfulness both at home and at work. These are practical techniques that don't require extra time; instead, they're about doing the things you're already doing, but with a more mindful approach.

Mindful Routines at Home

Home is where we often unwind, but it's also where we juggle endless to-dos. From cleaning to cooking, daily chores can feel repetitive or even stressful. By bringing mindfulness into these routines, we can turn them into moments of calm and focus.

1. Mindful Cleaning

Cleaning might not be your favourite activity, but it can be a surprisingly calming practice when done mindfully. Here's how to approach it:

1. **Set an intention**: Before you start, take a moment to appreciate the act of cleaning. Think of it as clearing both physical and mental space.
2. **Focus on each movement**: Notice the sensation of wiping a surface, the texture of the cloth, or the sound of scrubbing. Let your mind focus on these simple actions.
3. **Stay present**: If your mind starts to wander, gently bring your attention back to the task. Cleaning can become a meditative, grounding activity when we stay connected to it.

Mindful cleaning can help you appreciate the process and make the task feel less like a chore and more like a reset for both your home and mind.

2. Mindful Cooking and Eating

Eating and cooking are wonderful opportunities to practice mindfulness. When we're fully present with food, we can find joy and appreciation in even the simplest meal.

1. **Prepare with awareness**: As you chop vegetables or stir a pot, notice the colours, textures, and smells. Let yourself be fully engaged with each step of the process.

2. **Savour each bite**: When you sit down to eat, take a moment to pause. Appreciate the appearance of your meal before you take your first bite.
3. **Eat slowly**: Chew each bite thoroughly and notice the flavours, textures, and aromas. Eating mindfully can help you feel more satisfied and connected to your body.

Mindful eating isn't just about slowing down; it's about truly enjoying each moment of the experience.

3. A Mindful Start and End to Your Day

Bookending your day with mindfulness can bring a sense of calm to both morning and evening.

- **Morning**: Begin with a few deep breaths as you wake up. Notice how your body feels, take a moment to stretch, and set an intention for the day ahead.
- **Evening**: Before bed, spend a minute reflecting on something you're grateful for. Let this moment of gratitude help you unwind and close your day on a positive note.

These small moments don't take much time, but they can shift your mindset, making you feel more grounded and prepared for the day or relaxed for a restful night.

Mindfulness in the Workplace

The workplace can be one of the most challenging places to stay mindful. Between deadlines, meetings, and constant notifications, staying present can feel nearly impossible. But bringing mindfulness into work doesn't mean sitting in meditation all day — it's about finding small ways to stay focused, calm, and connected to your tasks and environment.

1. Mindful Focus with the "Single-Tasking" Approach

Multitasking is common in the workplace, but it can actually increase stress and make it harder to focus. Practicing mindfulness at work often starts with single-tasking or focusing on one task at a time.

1. **Choose one task to focus on**: Start with a task you can complete in a few minutes, like responding to an email or working on a project.
2. **Set a timer**: If you find it hard to stay focused, set a timer for 5-10 minutes and dedicate that time solely to the task at hand.
3. **Be fully present**: Let yourself dive into the task, noticing each step and detail without getting distracted by other thoughts.

Single-tasking can help reduce mental clutter and increase productivity, leaving you feeling more accomplished and less scattered.

2. Taking Mindful Breaks

Taking regular breaks is crucial for maintaining focus and preventing burnout. Even a quick, mindful break can refresh your mind and keep you going through the day.

1. **Step away from your workspace**: Go for a short walk, stretch, or simply sit somewhere quiet.
2. **Focus on your breath**: Use one of the breathing exercises from Chapter 3, like deep belly breathing, to reconnect with yourself.
3. **Observe your surroundings**: Take a few moments to notice something around you—whether it's a plant, a window view, or even a piece of art on the wall.

Taking just a few minutes to reset can help you feel more energised and better able to handle your next task.

3. Mindful Listening in Meetings

In a busy workplace, conversations can often feel rushed or shallow. Practicing mindful listening can help you connect with others and improve communication.

1. **Give full attention**: When someone is speaking, focus solely on their words. Try not to think about your response until they're done.
2. **Notice your reactions**: If you feel impatient or distracted, take a breath and bring your focus back to the person.
3. **Ask open questions**: Practicing mindfulness includes being curious. Ask follow-up questions that show genuine interest and help you better understand the other person's perspective.

Mindful listening not only strengthens relationships but also helps create a positive and collaborative work environment.

Setting Boundaries: Protecting Your Time and Energy

Mindfulness in both home and work life often involves setting healthy boundaries. When we're constantly "on," it's easy to become overwhelmed. Here are a few ways to set boundaries mindfully:

- **At Home**: Give yourself permission to take breaks, say no to activities when needed, and protect your time to recharge. Taking care of yourself is essential to being able to support others.
- **At Work**: Set clear limits on working hours and try to minimise after-hours tasks. If possible, communicate your needs openly with colleagues, letting them know when you're available and when you need time to focus.

Boundaries are a powerful way to practice mindfulness, reminding you that your well-being is a priority.

Mindfulness for a Balanced Life

Incorporating mindfulness into home and work routines isn't about adding extra time — it's about making each moment count. By practicing mindfulness in the things you're already doing, you create a sense of calm, balance, and intention that can make a big difference in your daily experience.

Over time, you'll likely find that mindfulness isn't just something you "do" but becomes part of how you approach life. When you're fully present, even the busiest days can feel a little lighter, and you're better equipped to handle whatever comes your way.

Chapter Reflection: Bringing Mindfulness into Your Day

How might you bring a bit more mindfulness to your home and work life. Are there any routines or tasks you could try doing mindfully? Is there one boundary you could set that would help you feel more balanced?

As you try out these practices, notice how they make you feel. These small moments of mindfulness may seem simple, but they can create a meaningful shift in how you experience your day.

Chapter 6: Managing Stress and Emotions Mindfully

Understanding Stress Responses

Stress is a part of life, and we all feel it from time to time. It can be triggered by work deadlines, personal relationships, or even

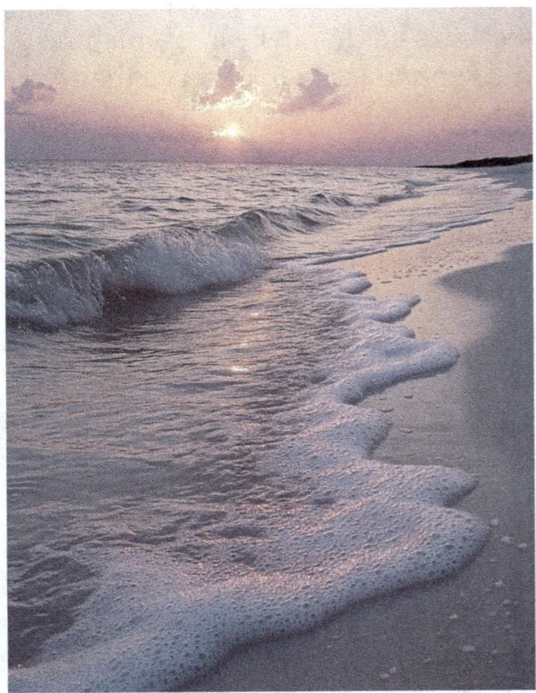

a crowded schedule. While stress itself isn't necessarily a bad thing, how we respond to it can make a big difference. When we're stressed, our bodies and minds react quickly, often pushing us into a "fight or flight" mode that's hard to control.

This is where mindfulness can help. Instead of getting swept away by stress, mindfulness gives us the tools to pause, take a breath, and respond thoughtfully. Mindfulness doesn't eliminate stress, but it can change how we experience it. By becoming more aware of our stress responses, we can learn to approach difficult moments with a sense of calm and control.

In this chapter, we'll explore practical exercises to help you notice and manage stress in a mindful way. These techniques are designed to be easy to incorporate into daily life, helping you stay grounded even in challenging situations.

Emotional Awareness Exercises

Emotions are part of what makes us human, and they can range from joy and excitement to sadness and frustration. Some emotions feel great, while others are more difficult to sit with. The practice of mindfulness teaches us that instead of pushing away or judging our emotions, we can learn to observe them with curiosity and compassion.

Here are a few exercises to help you practice emotional awareness, especially during times of stress.

1. Noticing and Naming Emotions

When we're in the middle of a strong emotion, it can feel overwhelming. One way to manage this is by simply acknowledging and naming what you're feeling.

1. **Pause and take a deep breath**: If you feel a strong emotion coming up, take a moment to stop and breathe.
2. **Name the emotion**: Quietly say to yourself, "I feel…" and then name the emotion, such as "angry," "anxious," or "sad."
3. **Acknowledge the feeling**: Instead of judging the emotion or trying to change it, just notice it. Remind yourself, "It's okay to feel this way."

Naming emotions helps us bring awareness to them without getting lost in them. It can feel surprisingly calming, as if you're stepping outside of the emotion and observing it rather than being consumed by it.

2. The "RAIN" Technique

This is a mindfulness technique that can be especially helpful for difficult emotions. RAIN stands for Recognise, Allow, Investigate, and Nurture.

1. **Recognise**: Notice what emotion is present. Simply recognise it without judgment.
2. **Allow**: Allow the emotion to be there, even if it's uncomfortable. Remind yourself that it's okay to feel what you're feeling.
3. **Investigate**: Gently explore the emotion. Ask yourself, "Where do I feel this in my body? What thoughts are coming up with this feeling?"
4. **Nurture**: Offer yourself kindness and compassion. Imagine what you would say to a friend who's feeling this way and offer those same words to yourself.

The RAIN technique can help you slow down and approach your emotions with care. It's a way to respond to difficult feelings rather than react to them, allowing you to feel more grounded and in control.

3. Practicing Self-Compassion

When we're feeling stressed or emotional, it's easy to be hard on ourselves. Practicing self-compassion can help us be kinder to ourselves in these moments.

1. **Place a hand on your heart**: This simple gesture can bring comfort and help you feel connected to yourself.
2. **Say something kind**: Choose a phrase that feels soothing, like "It's okay to feel this way" or "I'm doing the best I can."
3. **Breathe deeply**: Take a few deep breaths, letting each one remind you that you're here for yourself.

Self-compassion is about treating yourself with the same care you'd offer a friend. When you approach your emotions with kindness, you're more likely to feel calm and resilient.

Responding Instead of Reacting

Mindfulness teaches us to respond to stress and emotions rather than react impulsively. Reacting often means letting our emotions take over, leading to hasty decisions or words we might regret. Responding, on the other hand, means taking a moment to pause and choose how we want to proceed.

Steps to Practice Responding Mindfully:

1. **Pause and take a breath**: The first step to responding mindfully is creating space. Even a single deep breath can help you step back from the situation.
2. **Acknowledge the emotion**: Notice what you're feeling and name it, as we practiced earlier.
3. **Ask yourself, "What do I need right now?"**: This could be a moment of calm, a kind word to yourself, or even just a quick break. By asking what you need, you're focusing on a constructive response.
4. **Proceed with intention**: When you're ready, choose how you want to move forward. Responding with intention can help you feel more grounded and in control.

Responding instead of reacting gives you the power to handle stress with clarity. It's a skill that may take practice, but over time, it becomes easier to pause, breathe, and respond thoughtfully.

Using Breath to Calm the Body and Mind

As we explored in Chapter 3, the breath is a powerful tool for managing stress. When we're stressed, our breathing often becomes shallow and quick, which signals to our body that we're in danger. By practicing deep, mindful breathing, we can send the opposite signal — that we're safe and can relax.

Here's a quick breathing exercise to try whenever you feel stressed:

1. **Sit comfortably**: Place both feet on the floor and let your hands rest on your lap.
2. Take a slow, deep breath in through your nose: Feel your belly expand as you breathe in.
3. **Exhale slowly through your mouth**: Release the breath fully, noticing how it feels as you let go.
4. **Repeat for a few breaths**: Focus on each inhale and exhale, letting them slow down your body and mind.

This simple breathing exercise can be used anytime you feel stress rising. It's a reminder to return to the present moment and let go of tension.

Finding Balance with Regular Mindfulness Practices

Managing stress and emotions isn't about eliminating them — it's about finding balance. Regular mindfulness practices, even for just a few minutes each day, can help you feel more grounded and resilient.

Consider choosing one or two exercises from this chapter to practice regularly. Over time, you'll likely find that it becomes easier to stay calm and centred, even in challenging moments.

Embracing Emotions Without Judgment

One of the most powerful aspects of mindfulness is learning to approach emotions without judgment. Instead of labelling feelings as "good" or "bad," mindfulness encourages us to see emotions as part of the human experience. Every feeling is valid and worth acknowledging.

As you practice managing stress and emotions mindfully, remember that it's okay to feel whatever you feel. By approaching each emotion with openness and compassion, you can experience greater peace, even in the midst of life's ups and downs.

Chapter Reflection: Practicing Self-Compassion

As you finish this chapter, take time to reflect on how it felt to work with your emotions in a mindful way. Were there any techniques that felt especially helpful? How did it feel to acknowledge your emotions rather than push them away?

Note a few thoughts about your experience. Practicing self-compassion and responding mindfully to emotions is a journey, and each step you take helps you grow stronger, kinder, and more resilient.

Chapter 7: Practicing Self-Compassion and Kindness

What is Self-Compassion?

Self-compassion is simply the practice of being kind to ourselves. While it's often easy to show compassion toward others, we're not always as gentle with ourselves. Instead, we might be quick to criticise, judge, or blame ourselves when things go wrong. Practicing self-compassion means treating ourselves with the same understanding, patience, and kindness that we'd offer a friend.

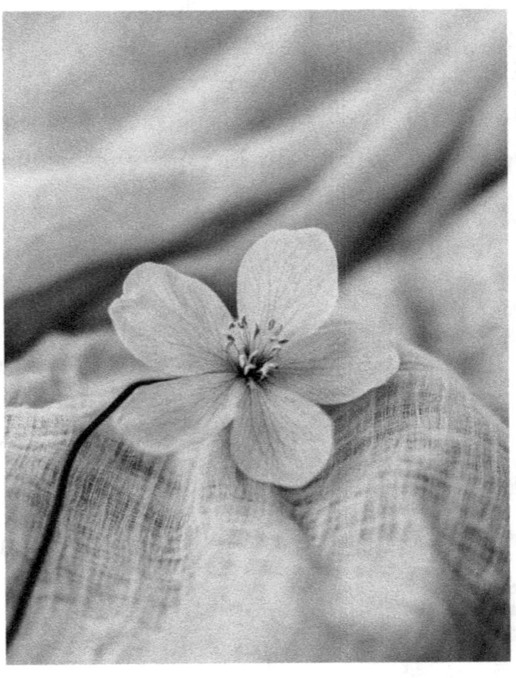

The truth is, self-compassion is a powerful tool for resilience and mental well-being. When we're kind to ourselves, we're better able to navigate stress and challenges. We become more forgiving, more adaptable, and, ultimately, more at peace.

In this chapter, we'll explore some simple practices to help you cultivate self-compassion and kindness in everyday life. These techniques are designed to help you build a more positive relationship with yourself, which in turn can strengthen your relationships with others.

The Benefits of Self-Compassion

Self-compassion isn't just a nice idea; it's backed by research as a source of strength and resilience. Studies show that people who practice self-compassion are better able to manage stress, cope with failure, and experience greater happiness overall.

Some of the benefits of self-compassion include:

- **Reduced Stress**: When we're kind to ourselves, we're less likely to dwell on mistakes or harshly criticise ourselves.
- **Greater Emotional Resilience**: Self-compassion can help us bounce back from setbacks and face challenges with a calm mind.
- **Improved Relationships**: The kindness we show to ourselves often extends to others, strengthening our connections.

Self-compassion doesn't mean avoiding responsibility or ignoring problems. Instead, it's about creating a supportive inner environment that helps us learn, grow, and find balance in life.

Self-Compassion Exercises

Here are a few simple exercises to help you practice self-compassion. These techniques can be used whenever you're feeling stressed, upset, or in need of a little kindness.

1. The Self-Compassion Break

This exercise is designed for moments when you're feeling overwhelmed or self-critical. It's a quick way to remind yourself to treat yourself with care.

1. **Pause and take a deep breath**: Close your eyes if it's comfortable, and take a deep, calming breath.
2. **Acknowledge your feelings**: Quietly say to yourself, "This is a moment of suffering." Recognise that what you're experiencing is difficult.
3. **Remind yourself that you're not alone**: Say, "Suffering is a part of life." This can help you remember that everyone has struggles, and you're not alone in feeling this way.
4. **Offer kindness to yourself**: Place a hand on your heart or another comforting gesture, and say, "May I be kind to myself." Choose any words that feel supportive, like "I'm doing the best I can."

The Self-Compassion Break helps us pause, acknowledge our experience, and offer ourselves the same care we'd give to a friend. It's a simple way to remember that it's okay to feel what we're feeling.

2. Writing a Kind Letter to Yourself

Writing a letter to yourself can be a powerful way to practice self-compassion, especially during challenging times.

1. **Think of a difficult situation**: Choose a situation where you're struggling or feeling self-critical.
2. **Write with kindness**: Imagine that you're writing to a friend going through the same experience. Use gentle, understanding language, and express empathy for what you're feeling.
3. **Offer words of support**: End the letter with some encouraging words, reminding yourself that you're not alone and that it's okay to feel this way.

Writing a compassionate letter can help you gain perspective and see your situation with more understanding. Keep the letter and reread it whenever you need a reminder to be kind to yourself.

Our inner dialogue plays a big role in how we feel about ourselves. Practicing positive self-talk means choosing to speak to ourselves with kindness rather than criticism.

1. **Notice negative thoughts**: When you catch yourself thinking something negative about yourself, pause and take a deep breath.
2. **Reframe with kindness**: Replace the negative thought with a kinder, more balanced statement. For example, change "I always mess up" to "It's okay to make mistakes. I'm learning and doing my best."
3. **Practice regularly**: The more you practice positive self-talk, the easier it becomes to be kind to yourself in difficult moments.

Positive self-talk isn't about ignoring challenges but about being supportive and gentle with ourselves. Over time, it can make a big difference in how we view ourselves and our experiences.

Practicing Kindness Toward Others

Self-compassion often extends naturally to others. When we're kind to ourselves, it's easier to show kindness to the people around us. Practicing kindness toward others doesn't have to be grand or complicated—small gestures of compassion can have a big impact.

1. Mindful Listening

One of the simplest ways to show kindness is to listen mindfully when someone is speaking.

- **Give your full attention**: Focus on the person's words and avoid thinking about your response while they're talking.
- **Show empathy**: Nod, smile, or use small words of encouragement to show that you're listening.
- **Avoid judgment**: Try to listen without judging or assuming. Mindful listening helps build connection and shows others that they matter.

2. Practicing Gratitude for Others

Gratitude is a powerful form of kindness that we can offer to others. This practice helps us focus on the positive qualities of the people in our lives.

1. **Think of someone you appreciate**: Take a moment to think of a family member, friend, or colleague.
2. **List three things you're grateful for**: Silently list three things you appreciate about this person.
3. **Express your gratitude**: If possible, share your gratitude with them—whether it's through a text, a call, or in person.

Practicing gratitude for others strengthens our relationships and helps us see the good in those around us.

Building a Habit of Kindness

Practicing kindness and self-compassion isn't a one-time event; it's something we can cultivate every day. Here are a few ways to make kindness a regular part of your life:

- **Start with small acts**: Kindness doesn't have to be complicated. Holding the door, offering a genuine compliment, or sending a quick thank-you note can make a difference.
- **Be kind to yourself every morning**: Begin each day with a small act of self-kindness. Take a moment to appreciate yourself and acknowledge that you're doing your best.
- **Practice forgiving yourself**: When you make a mistake, take a deep breath and remind yourself that it's okay. Let go of harsh judgments and embrace self-forgiveness.

Building kindness into daily life helps us create a positive, supportive environment for ourselves and those around us. It's a simple but powerful way to make each day a little brighter.

Embracing Imperfection

Practicing self-compassion means accepting that we're all imperfect. Perfection isn't the goal of mindfulness or self-kindness; rather, it's about embracing ourselves as we are, with all our strengths and flaws. Life isn't always easy, but we can choose to approach it with kindness, both toward ourselves and others.

Remember, each small act of self-compassion is a step toward greater resilience and happiness. When you're kind to yourself, you're better able to handle life's challenges with grace.

Chapter Reflection: Building Your Kindness Practice

Take a moment to think about how you might bring more kindness and self-compassion into your daily life. Are there any self-compassion exercises that felt especially meaningful? How does it feel to treat yourself with kindness?

If you'd like, jot down some thoughts on your experience. Practicing kindness is a journey, and each small act of self-compassion brings you closer to a more balanced, fulfilling life.

Chapter 8: Mindful Relationships

Why Mindfulness Matters in Relationships

Relationships are one of the most fulfilling parts of life, but they can also be a source of stress, misunderstanding, and even 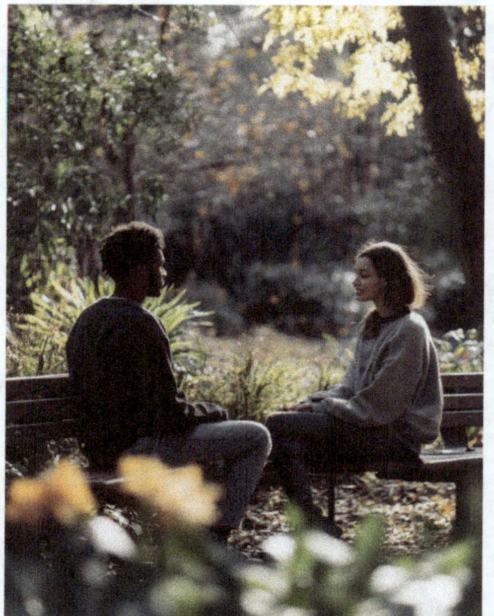 frustration. Whether it's with family, friends, colleagues, or partners, maintaining healthy, meaningful relationships takes effort. Mindfulness can help us connect more deeply with others, bringing empathy, patience, and presence into our interactions.

When we're fully present with someone, we're able to listen more deeply, communicate more openly, and respond with compassion rather than reacting out of habit or frustration. In this chapter, we'll explore ways to bring mindfulness into your relationships, helping you create stronger, more authentic connections.

Listening Mindfully

Mindful listening is one of the most powerful ways to show care and respect in any relationship. Often, when someone is speaking, we're only half listening — our minds may wander, or we might be busy planning our response. When we listen mindfully, however, we focus entirely on the person in front of us, giving them our full attention.

Steps for Mindful Listening:

1. **Set an intention to be present**: Before a conversation, take a deep breath and set the intention to fully listen to the other person.
2. **Focus on their words**: Let go of any urge to interrupt, judge, or plan your response. Simply listen to the words they're saying.
3. **Notice non-verbal cues**: Pay attention to body language, tone of voice, and facial expressions. These can give you clues about how the other person is feeling.
4. **Reflect back**: When they finish, reflect back what you heard to show that you're listening. This could be a simple statement like, "It sounds like you're feeling…" or "I hear that you're saying…"

Mindful listening is a gift you can give to anyone, helping them feel seen, heard, and valued. It's also a practice that naturally brings you into the present moment, grounding you in the here and now.

Responding with Empathy

Empathy is the ability to understand and share the feelings of another. In mindful relationships, empathy allows us to connect with others on a deeper level, especially when they're going through a difficult time. Mindful empathy involves pausing, taking a step back, and doing our best to see things from the other person's perspective.

Practicing Empathy in Conversations:

1. **Pause before responding**: When someone shares something difficult, pause for a moment before you respond. This gives you a chance to process their words and respond thoughtfully.
2. **Acknowledge their feelings**: Even if you don't fully understand, acknowledge the other person's feelings. You could say something like, "I can see that this is really hard for you," or "I understand that you're feeling upset."
3. **Avoid judgment**: Empathy means setting aside your own judgments or opinions. Focus on simply being there for the person and offering them a safe space to share.

When we respond with empathy, we show that we're truly present and care about their experience. Empathy deepens relationships and fosters mutual understanding and trust.

Practicing Non-Judgment

It's natural to have opinions, but in mindful relationships, practicing non-judgment can be a powerful tool for building understanding and connection. When we judge, we close ourselves off from fully accepting the other person. By letting go of judgment, we make space for open-mindedness and acceptance.

Tips for Practicing Non-Judgment:

1. **Notice your reactions**: When you feel a judgmental thought coming up, pause and take a breath. Simply notice the thought without acting on it.
2. **Focus on understanding**: Shift your attention from judging to understanding. Ask yourself, "What can I learn from this person's perspective?"
3. **Practice acceptance**: Remember that everyone has their own journey and experiences. Practice accepting the person as they are, without needing them to change.

Non-judgment doesn't mean you have to agree with everything someone says. It simply means respecting their right to their own feelings and experiences.

Building Deeper Connections with Mindful Presence

True connection happens when we're fully present with another person. By bringing mindfulness into your relationships, you can create more moments of real connection. Here are some ways to practice mindful presence in your relationships.

1. Make Eye Contact

Eye contact is a simple but powerful way to show that you're fully engaged. When you're talking with someone, try to maintain gentle eye contact. This shows that you're listening and helps you stay focused on the person in front of you.

2. Use Positive Body Language

Our body language says a lot about how we're feeling. Use open, relaxed body language to signal that you're present and receptive. Avoid crossing your arms or looking away frequently, as these can make you seem closed off.

3. Offer Small Gestures of Kindness

Kindness is an essential part of mindful relationships. Small gestures, like a warm smile, a kind word, or a gentle touch, can make someone feel cared for and valued. These small acts of kindness create positive energy and help strengthen your connections.

Handling Conflict Mindfully

Conflict is a natural part of any relationship, but mindfulness can help us handle it with calm and respect. When we approach conflict mindfully, we're less likely to say or do things we might regret. Instead, we can communicate our needs and feelings in a way that builds understanding.

Steps to Handle Conflict Mindfully:

1. **Pause before reacting**: If you feel angry or upset, take a moment to pause and breathe before you respond. This short break can help you cool down and approach the situation with a clear mind.
2. **Express your feelings calmly**: Use "I" statements to share your feelings without blaming the other person. For example, "I feel hurt when…" or "I need…"
3. **Listen to their perspective**: Allow the other person to share their side and try to listen without interrupting. Show empathy and understanding, even if you don't agree.

4. **Focus on finding a solution**: Approach the conflict with a willingness to find a solution that works for both of you. Remember that the goal is mutual understanding, not "winning" the argument.

Handling conflict mindfully helps you communicate more effectively and strengthens trust in your relationships.

Practicing Gratitude in Relationships

Gratitude is a simple but powerful way to deepen connections with others. When we practice gratitude, we focus on the positive qualities of the people in our lives, which helps us appreciate and value them.

Daily Gratitude Practice:

1. **Choose one person**: Think of someone in your life, whether it's a friend, family member, or colleague.
2. **List three things you appreciate**: Silently or out loud, list three things you're grateful for about this person. It could be their kindness, their sense of humour, or the support they give you.
3. **Express your gratitude**: If possible, let the person know what you appreciate about them. A simple "thank you" or "I appreciate you" can go a long way.

Gratitude not only improves relationships but also boosts our own happiness and well-being. When we appreciate others, we create a more positive and supportive environment for ourselves and those around us.

Embracing Imperfection in Relationships

Relationships aren't always easy, and they don't need to be perfect to be meaningful. Embracing imperfection means accepting that misunderstandings, disagreements, and challenges are natural parts of connecting with others. Mindfulness helps us navigate these moments with patience and compassion, allowing us to grow and learn together.

Remember, being mindful in relationships is a practice, not a destination. Each moment of kindness, empathy, and presence builds a foundation of trust and connection. Over time, these mindful interactions create relationships that are rich, supportive, and deeply fulfilling.

Chapter Reflection: Nurturing Mindful Connections

Reflect on your relationships and how you might bring more mindfulness into them. Is there someone you'd like to listen to more deeply? Or perhaps a small act of kindness you could share with someone close to you?

As you explore these practices, remember that building mindful relationships is a journey. Each small step brings you closer to meaningful, genuine connections with the people in your life.

Chapter 9: Mindfulness on the Go

Bringing Mindfulness into Busy Moments

Mindfulness doesn't have to be limited to quiet spaces or specific routines. In fact, some of the best opportunities to practice mindfulness are during life's busier moments. Whether you're commuting, standing in line, or taking a quick break between tasks, these small pauses throughout the day can help you feel more balanced and present, no matter how hectic things get.

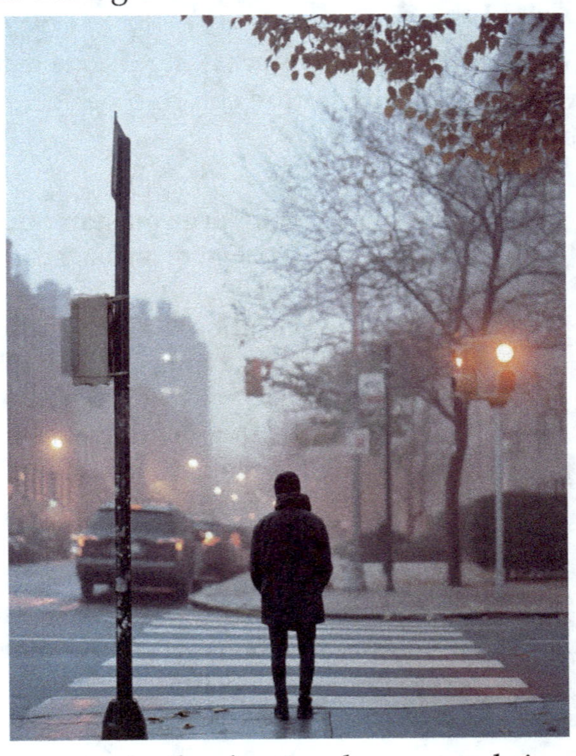

In this chapter, we'll explore easy, portable mindfulness practices that can fit into even the busiest days. These techniques don't require any special setup or tools; they're simple ways to bring calm, focus, and presence to whatever you're doing, wherever you are.

Incorporating Mindfulness in Daily Life

Mindfulness on the go is about turning everyday activities into opportunities for awareness and grounding. Here are a few easy ways to practice mindfulness in moments that are already part of your routine.

1. Mindful Commuting

Whether you're driving, taking public transport, or even walking, your commute can be a perfect time to practice mindfulness.

1. **Set an intention before you start**: Before beginning your commute, take a deep breath and set an intention to stay present.
2. **Focus on the sensations**: Notice the feeling of the steering wheel, the sounds around you, or the rhythm of your steps. Let your senses ground you in the moment.
3. **Observe without judgment**: If you get stuck in traffic or experience delays, notice any feelings of impatience or frustration. Acknowledge them without judgment, and gently bring your focus back to the present.

Mindful commuting helps transform a potentially stressful time into a moment of calm, allowing you to arrive at your destination feeling more centred.

2. Waiting in Line with Awareness

Waiting is a part of life, but it doesn't have to feel like wasted time. Use these moments as a chance to pause, reset, and reconnect with yourself.

1. **Stand with awareness**: Notice how you're standing and allow yourself to relax any areas of tension in your body.

2. **Focus on your breath**: Take slow, gentle breaths, letting each inhale and exhale bring you back to the present.
3. **Observe your surroundings**: Look around and notice details you might usually overlook—the colours, shapes, or sounds around you.

This practice can help you feel more patient and grounded, turning a routine wait into a peaceful moment of mindfulness.

3. Taking a Mini Mindful Break

Throughout the day, take short, mindful breaks to reset your mind and body. These breaks don't need to be long; even a minute or two can make a difference.

1. **Pause what you're doing**: Stop your activity and take a deep breath.
2. **Notice how you feel**: Check in with yourself and notice if there's any tension, tiredness, or stress.
3. **Take three mindful breaths**: With each breath, let go of any tension and allow yourself to feel more relaxed.

A mini mindful break is a quick way to refresh your energy and return to your tasks with a clear mind. Try to take these breaks every couple of hours, or whenever you feel the need to reset.

Portable Mindfulness Practices

Here are a few more techniques you can use anytime, anywhere, to bring mindfulness into your day.

1. The "STOP" Practice

This is a quick exercise that you can do whenever you feel stressed or overwhelmed. It's called the "STOP" practice, and it stands for Stop, Take a breath, Observe, and Proceed.

1. **S – Stop**: Whatever you're doing, pause for a moment.
2. **T – Take a breath**: Take a slow, deep breath, allowing yourself to relax.
3. **O – Observe**: Notice what's happening around you and within you. Are you feeling stressed? Calm? Just observe.
4. **P – Proceed**: Continue with your activity, bringing this sense of awareness with you.

The STOP practice is a simple way to reset and refocus, helping you respond to situations with clarity rather than reacting automatically.

2. 5-4-3-2-1 Grounding Technique

This exercise is especially helpful if you're feeling stressed, anxious, or overwhelmed. It uses your senses to bring you back to the present moment.

1. **Notice five things you can see**: Look around and take in your surroundings.
2. **Notice four things you can touch**: Feel the texture of your clothing, a surface nearby, or an object in your hand.
3. **Notice three things you can hear**: Listen for sounds you might not usually notice.
4. **Notice two things you can smell**: If possible, notice any scents around you.
5. **Notice one thing you can taste**: If you have a drink or snack nearby, take a sip or bite and savour it.

The 5-4-3-2-1 technique can quickly ground you in the present and calm your mind during times of stress or anxiety.

3. The Mindful Hand Exercise

This is a discreet mindfulness practice you can do anytime to bring your focus back to the present.

1. **Place your hands together**: Close your eyes and feel the sensation of your hands touching.
2. **Focus on the details**: Notice the temperature, the texture of your skin, and the pressure between your hands.
3. **Take a few deep breaths**: With each breath, focus on the feeling of your hands. Let this simple sensation bring you into the moment.

The mindful hand exercise is subtle and grounding, offering a quick way to centre yourself without drawing attention to the fact that you're practicing mindfulness.

Mindfulness Apps and Tools

If you find it helpful, there are plenty of apps and tools available that can support your mindfulness practice on the go. Many apps offer short, guided meditations, breathing exercises, and reminders to pause throughout the day.

Some popular mindfulness apps include:

- **Headspace**: Offers guided meditations for various situations, including stress, focus, and relaxation.
- **Calm**: Features guided sessions, breathing exercises, and soothing sounds to help with mindfulness.
- **Insight Timer**: Provides free guided meditations, music, and tools for mindfulness on the go.

Using an app can help you incorporate mindfulness into your daily routine, especially when you're busy and need a little extra support.

Building a Habit of Portable Mindfulness

Making mindfulness a part of your daily life doesn't have to be complicated. Here are a few tips for building a habit of mindfulness on the go:

1. **Use everyday moments**: Practice mindfulness during activities you already do, like walking, commuting, or waiting in line.
2. **Set reminders**: Use a gentle alarm or phone notification to remind yourself to pause and take a mindful breath every few hours.
3. **Be flexible**: Don't worry if you can't practice every day. Mindfulness is about being present, so just do what feels right in the moment.

The goal of portable mindfulness is to help you feel grounded, centred, and connected, no matter where you are or what you're doing.

Finding Calm in a Busy World

Life is full of moments where we feel rushed, stressed, or distracted. Portable mindfulness gives us the chance to slow down, even for a few seconds, and reconnect with ourselves. These small practices might seem simple, but they can have a big impact on your overall sense of well-being.

By bringing mindfulness into your everyday activities, you create a calm centre within yourself that you can return to anytime you need it. Over time, you'll find that it becomes easier to stay present and peaceful, no matter how busy life gets.

Chapter Reflection: Practicing Mindfulness on the Go

Take a moment to reflect on the techniques in this chapter. Which practice do you think would fit best into your daily routine? Are there any specific moments in your day where you could pause, breathe, and bring yourself back to the present?

As you try out these techniques, remember that mindfulness is a journey. Each moment you spend practicing is a step toward greater balance and peace in your daily life.

Chapter 10: Sustaining Your Practice

Why Sustaining Your Mindfulness Practice Matters

Starting a mindfulness practice is a powerful step but keeping it going is what brings lasting benefits. Like any new habit,

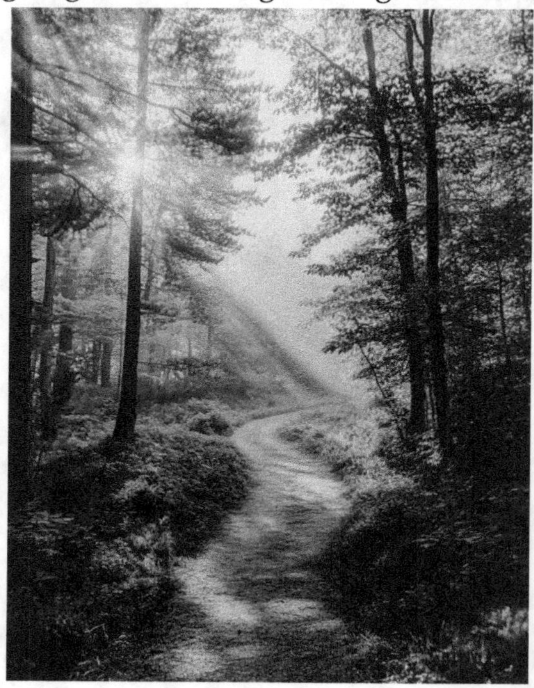

mindfulness is something that becomes more natural with time and consistency. The more you practice, the more it weaves into your life, creating a strong foundation for inner calm, resilience, and clarity.

Sustaining a mindfulness practice doesn't mean striving for perfection or practicing for hours every day. It's about finding a rhythm that works for you, one that allows mindfulness to be a gentle, supportive presence in your life. In this chapter, we'll explore ways to keep your practice going, overcome common challenges, and deepen your connection to mindfulness over time.

Overcoming Common Challenges

Maintaining a mindfulness practice isn't always easy. Life can get busy, motivation can wane, and distractions are everywhere. Here are some common challenges and tips for working through them.

1. "I Don't Have Enough Time"

One of the biggest obstacles to a consistent mindfulness practice is feeling like there's not enough time. However, mindfulness doesn't require long sessions to be effective. Even a few minutes can make a difference.

- **Start small**: Aim for just 1-5 minutes each day, especially if you're short on time. Remember that mindfulness is about quality, not quantity.
- **Incorporate mindfulness into daily tasks**: Try bringing mindfulness into everyday activities, like eating, brushing your teeth, or commuting. This way, you're practicing without needing extra time.

2. "I Keep Forgetting to Practice"

Building any new habit takes time, and it's natural to forget. The key is to create small reminders that help you remember to pause and be mindful.

- **Use reminders**: Set a gentle reminder on your phone or write a small note to yourself as a visual cue.
- **Pair mindfulness with routines**: Attach your practice to something you already do daily, like drinking your morning coffee or washing the dishes. This helps make it a regular part of your routine.

3. "My Mind Won't Stop Wandering"

It's perfectly normal for the mind to wander, especially when you're starting out. Mindfulness isn't about stopping thoughts; it's about noticing them and gently guiding your attention back.

- **Be patient**: Instead of trying to fight your thoughts, simply observe them without judgment. Let each thought pass like a cloud drifting by in the sky.
- **Refocus with your breath**: Whenever you notice your mind wandering, take a deep breath and gently return your focus to the present.

Building a Personal Mindfulness Routine

To make mindfulness a sustainable part of your life, try creating a routine that suits your schedule and needs. Your routine doesn't need to be rigid or complicated; it's about finding what feels comfortable and achievable.

1. Start with a Small, Consistent Practice

Choose a manageable length of time that you can practice daily. This might be just five minutes in the morning or a few deep breaths before bed. The key is consistency, even if the practice is short.

2. Gradually Add More Time (If You'd Like)

Once your practice feels established, you may find that you want to extend it. Add a few minutes here and there, but only if it feels right. There's no pressure to have a long practice for it to be effective.

3. Explore Different Types of Mindfulness

As you get more comfortable, try exploring different types of mindfulness practices. You could experiment with mindful walking, guided meditations, body scans, or gratitude journalling. Variety can keep your practice engaging and help you discover what resonates most with you.

Deepening Your Connection to Mindfulness

As your mindfulness practice develops, you might find that you want to go a bit deeper. Here are a few ideas for strengthening your practice and gaining a deeper sense of peace and presence.

1. Journalling Your Experiences

Keeping a mindfulness journal can be a great way to reflect on your practice. Write down your observations, challenges, and any insights you gain along the way. This can help you track your progress and notice subtle changes in how you respond to life's ups and downs.

2. Practicing Gratitude Regularly

Gratitude and mindfulness go hand in hand. By focusing on what you're grateful for, you can deepen your sense of appreciation for the present moment. Consider adding a daily gratitude practice, where you write down three things you're thankful for each day.

3. Connecting with a Mindfulness Community

Practicing mindfulness with others can provide support, motivation, and new perspectives. Look for local mindfulness groups, online communities, or classes that align with your interests. Being part of a community can remind you that you're not alone in your journey and offer fresh insights.

Bringing Mindfulness into Challenging Times

Life is full of unexpected challenges, and it's during these times that mindfulness can be particularly valuable. When you're going through a difficult period, use mindfulness to stay grounded and connected to yourself.

1. Taking It One Day at a Time

During tough times, focus on taking things one day—or even one moment—at a time. When challenges feel overwhelming, bring your attention to the present and trust that you can handle each moment as it comes.

2. Using Breath as an Anchor

When stress or emotions feel overwhelming, turn to your breath as an anchor. A few deep breaths can provide comfort and a sense of control, helping you stay grounded.

3. Practicing Self-Compassion

Be kind to yourself, especially during difficult moments. Use the self-compassion techniques from Chapter 7, reminding yourself that it's okay to struggle and that you're doing your best. Self-compassion can help you find strength and resilience in even the hardest times.

Embracing Mindfulness as a Lifelong Journey

Mindfulness is not a destination; it's a journey. There's no "end" to mindfulness, no point at which you've learned it all or mastered every technique. Instead, mindfulness is something you carry with you throughout life, adapting it to fit your needs as you grow and change.

Over time, you'll likely find that mindfulness becomes a natural part of who you are, influencing the way you experience life, respond to challenges, and connect with others. Embrace this journey with curiosity and openness, allowing mindfulness to evolve alongside you.

Looking Forward: Continuing Your Practice

As you reach the end of this book, remember that your mindfulness journey is just beginning. Each day offers a new opportunity to practice, whether it's through mindful breathing, observing your surroundings, or simply being kind to yourself. Continue to explore, experiment, and let mindfulness support you in whatever ways feel meaningful.

Final Reflection: Your Mindfulness Journey

Take a moment to reflect on what you've learned and experienced throughout this journey. How has mindfulness made a difference in your life? Are there any practices you'd like to continue or deepen? Perhaps you'd like to set an intention for your mindfulness journey moving forward.

Remember, mindfulness is here to support you, no matter where you are in life. It's a gift you can always come back to, helping you find peace, presence, and balance in a busy world.

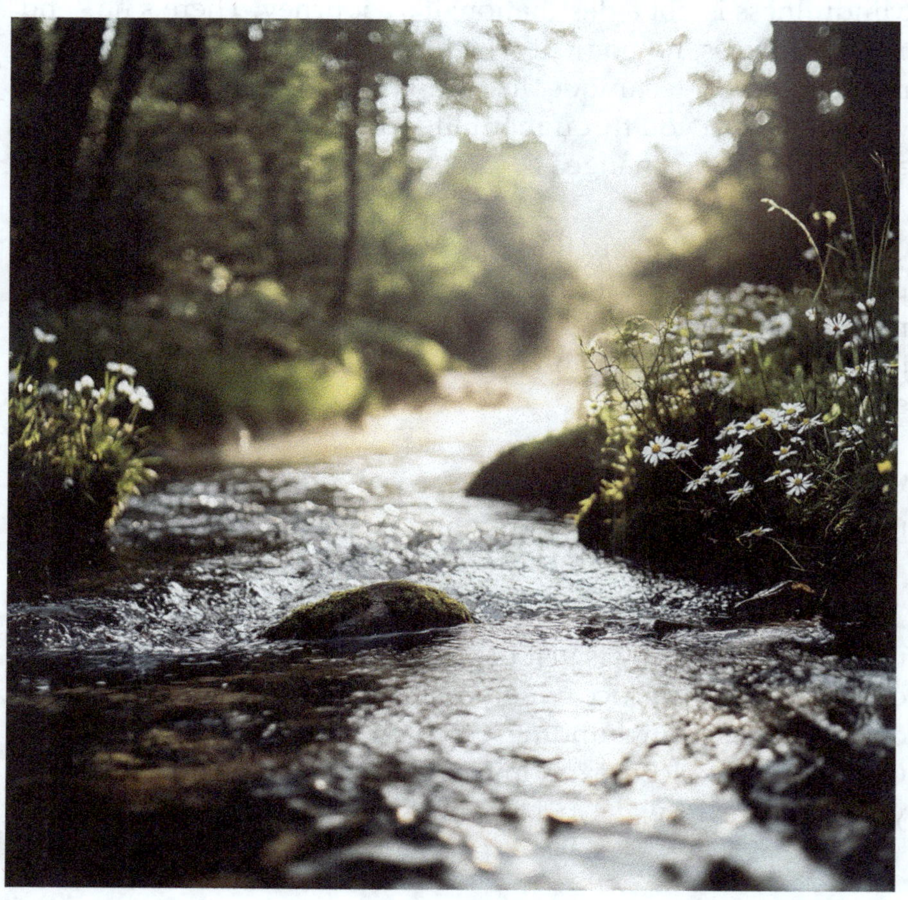

Appendices

Appendix A: Guided Mindfulness Practices

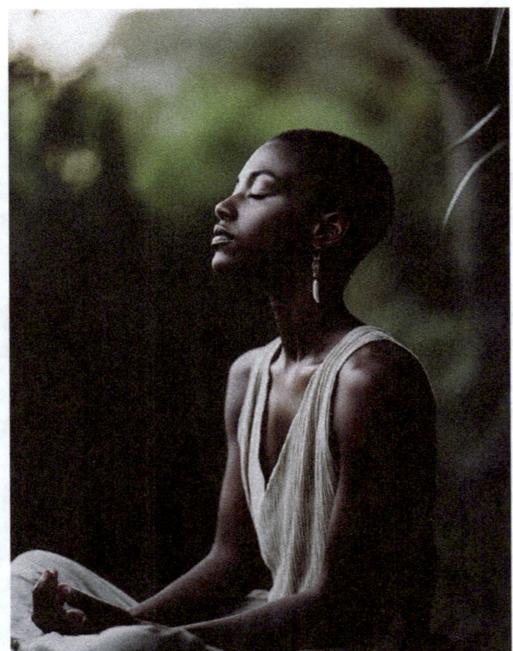

To make it easy for you to continue your mindfulness journey, here are some guided practices from the book that you can use anytime. Each practice is designed to be simple, accessible, and adaptable to fit your needs. These can be especially helpful if you're just starting out or if you're looking for a structured way to bring mindfulness into your day.

1. Breathing in Awareness

Use this exercise to connect with your breath whenever you need a moment of calm.

1. **Sit comfortably**: Settle into a position that feels easy, with both feet on the floor if you're seated.
2. **Take a deep breath in**: Breathe in slowly through your nose, feeling the air fill your lungs.
3. **Exhale fully**: Release the breath gently through your mouth.

4. **Notice the breath**: Continue breathing naturally and focus on the sensation of each inhale and exhale.
5. **Repeat for a few minutes**: If your mind wanders, gently bring it back to the breath.

2. The Five Senses Check-In

This practice can ground you in the present using your senses, making it perfect for times when you feel scattered or stressed.

1. **Take a deep breath**: Let yourself pause for a moment.
2. **Notice five things you can see**: Look around and observe the colours, shapes, or objects around you.
3. **Notice four things you can touch**: Feel the texture of your clothes, a nearby surface, or an object.
4. **Notice three things you can hear**: Listen for sounds in your environment, even the subtle ones.
5. **Notice two things you can smell**: Take note of any scents in the air, whether they're familiar or new.
6. **Notice one thing you can taste**: If you have something to sip or nibble, notice the taste. Otherwise, focus on the taste in your mouth.

3. The Self-Compassion Break

Use this exercise during difficult moments to remind yourself to treat yourself with kindness and understanding.

1. **Pause and take a breath**: Acknowledge what you're feeling and remind yourself that it's okay.
2. **Recognise the moment of struggle**: Silently say, "This is a moment of suffering."
3. **Remind yourself of common humanity**: Say, "Suffering is a part of life," to remember that you're not alone.
4. **Offer kindness to yourself**: Place a hand over your heart and say, "May I be kind to myself" or "I'm doing the best I can."

4. The STOP Practice

This is a quick way to centre yourself when you're feeling overwhelmed.

1. **S – Stop**: Pause whatever you're doing.
2. **T – Take a breath**: Take a slow, mindful breath to centre yourself.
3. **O – Observe**: Notice what's happening within and around you, without judgment.
4. **P – Proceed**: Continue with your activity, bringing this awareness with you.

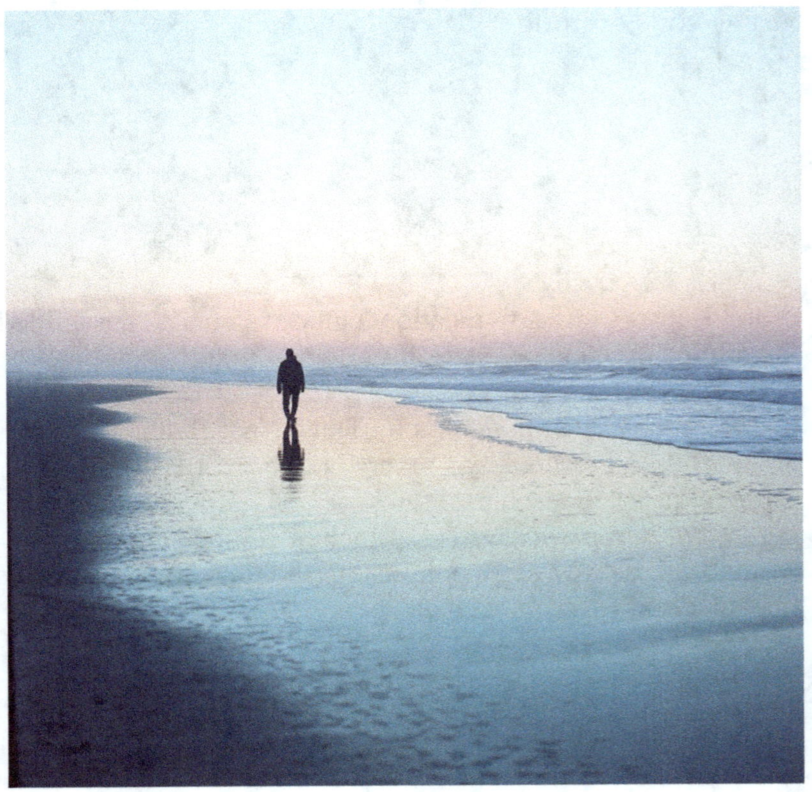

Appendix B: Further Reading and Resources

If you'd like to explore mindfulness further, here are some recommended books, apps, and resources that offer valuable guidance. These resources can help deepen your understanding and provide additional support as you continue your practice.

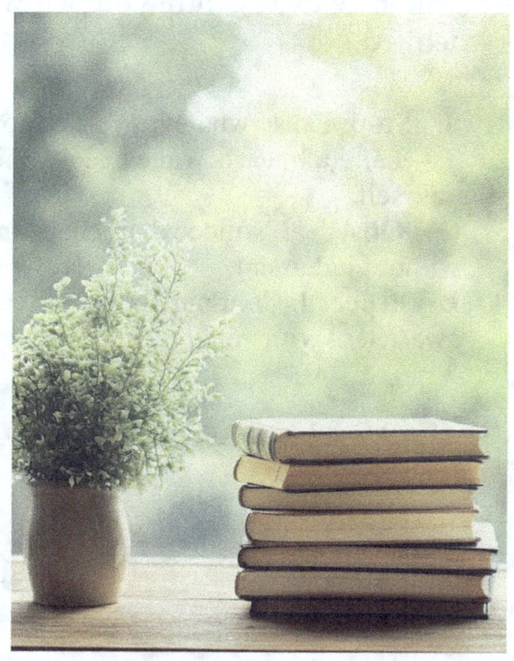

Books

- *Wherever You Go, There You Are* by Jon Kabat-Zinn: A foundational guide to mindfulness, filled with insights and practices for bringing mindfulness into everyday life.
- *The Miracle of Mindfulness* by Thich Nhat Hanh: A classic on mindfulness, written by a revered teacher, offering simple techniques and teachings.
- *Radical Acceptance* by Tara Brach: This book combines mindfulness with self-compassion, showing how to embrace yourself fully, even in challenging times.

Apps

- **Headspace**: A user-friendly app offering guided meditations for all levels, including short practices for busy moments.
- **Calm**: Known for its variety of mindfulness and sleep content, Calm offers guided meditations, breathing exercises, and calming music.

- **Insight Timer**: This app features thousands of free guided meditations, timers, and community features to support mindfulness.

Websites

- **Mindful.org**: A site dedicated to all things mindfulness, offering articles, guided practices, and resources for mindfulness in everyday life.
- **Centre for Mindful Self-Compassion**: A resourceful website with articles, exercises, and workshops on self-compassion, developed by Dr. Kristin Neff and Dr. Chris Germer.
- **Greater Good Science Centre (ggsc.berkeley.edu)**: A site offering research-based articles and practices for mindfulness, compassion, and emotional well-being.

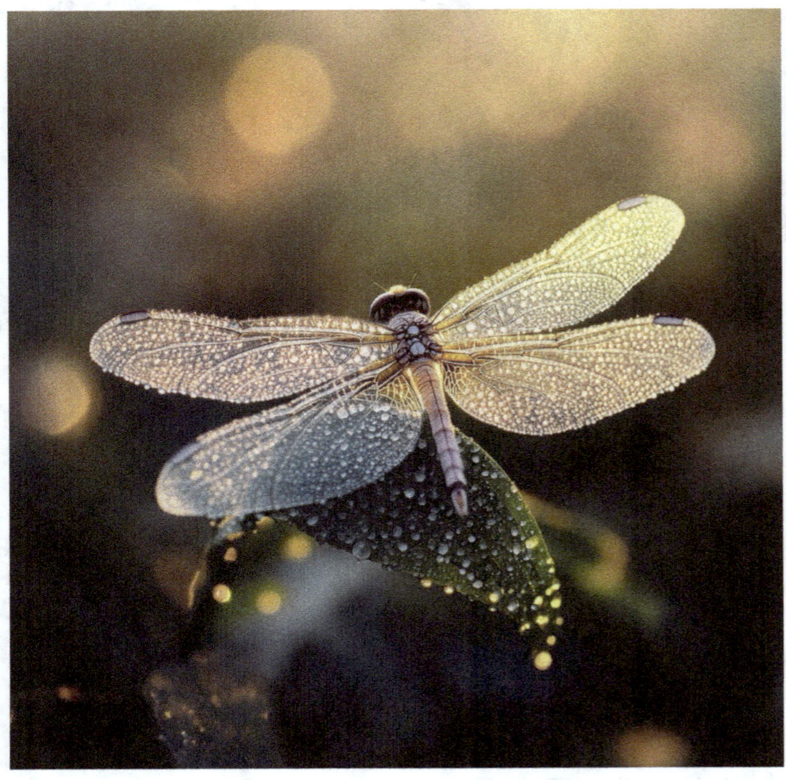

Appendix C: Beginner's Mindfulness Journal Template

Journalling can be a powerful way to reflect on your

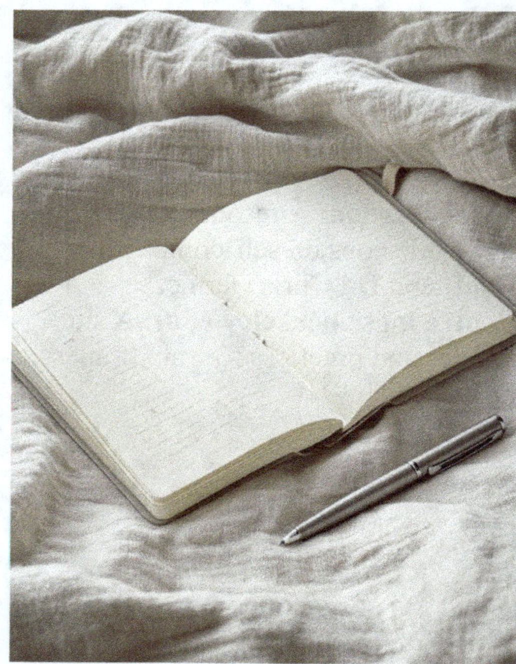

mindfulness journey, track your progress, and gain insights into your experiences. Use this template to start your own mindfulness journal, capturing your thoughts, feelings, and any changes you notice over time.

1. Daily Mindfulness Reflection

Use this simple prompt to check in with yourself at the end of each day.

- **Today, I practiced mindfulness by…**: Write down how you practiced mindfulness, whether it was a breathing exercise, mindful eating, or a short pause.
- **During my practice, I noticed…**: Reflect on anything you observed, whether it was your thoughts, emotions, or sensations in the body.
- **Today, I am grateful for…**: List one or two things you're grateful for today, helping to cultivate a sense of appreciation.

2. Weekly Reflection Questions

At the end of each week, use these questions to review and reflect on your experiences.

- What mindfulness practices felt most helpful this week?

- Did I face any challenges with mindfulness? If so, how did I handle them?
- How has mindfulness impacted my stress, emotions, or relationships this week?
- What am I learning about myself through my mindfulness practice?

3. Monthly Check-In

Once a month, take some time to look back on your mindfulness journey and set an intention for the month ahead.

- What positive changes have I noticed since starting mindfulness?
- How has my perspective on mindfulness or self-compassion changed?
- What area of mindfulness would I like to explore further next month?

Keeping a mindfulness journal helps create a record of your progress, showing you how far you've come and inspiring you to continue. Remember, there's no "right" way to journal—this is a personal space for reflection, discovery, and growth.

Closing Thoughts

Mindfulness is a lifelong journey, one that grows and evolves with you. Whether you're new to the practice or have been exploring it for some time, each step brings you closer to a sense of peace, balance, and presence. Use these appendices as tools to support you, offering gentle guidance as you continue on your path.

Thank you for joining this journey into mindfulness. May these practices bring you calm, clarity, and a deep connection to the present moment, wherever you are in life.

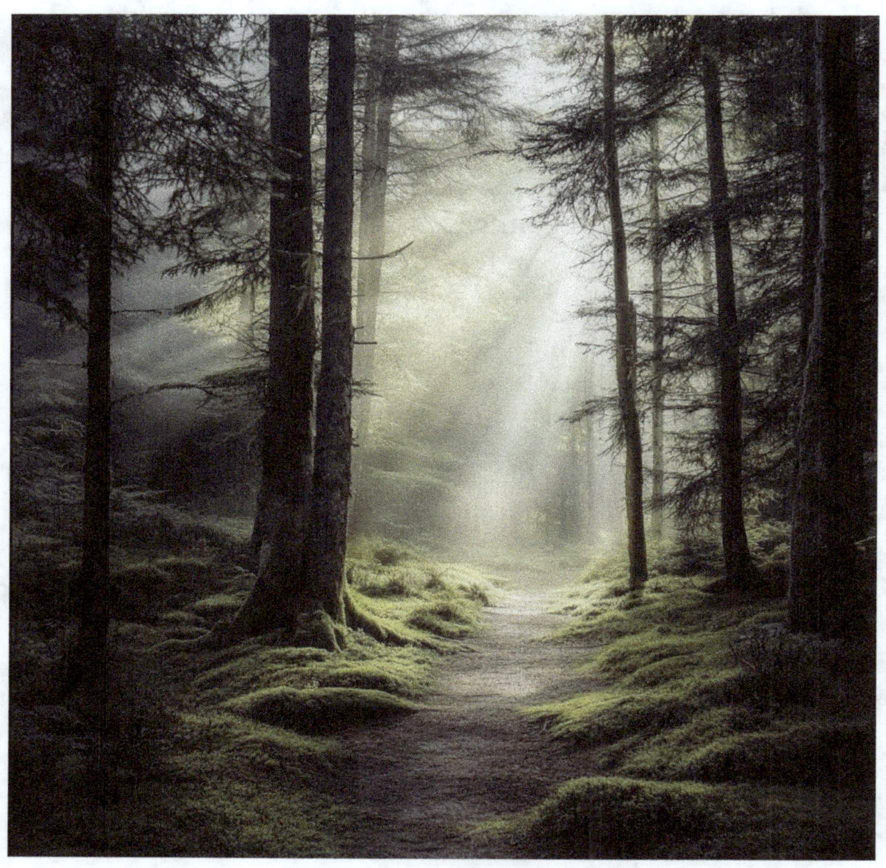